Cássia Marques da Rocha Hoelz
Taís Lopes Saranholi
Luciana P. F. Abbade

Nurses' Knowledge and Practice of Wounds

Cássia Marques da Rocha Hoelz
Taís Lopes Saranholi
Luciana P. F. Abbade

Nurses' Knowledge and Practice of Wounds

A cross-sectional study

ScienciaScripts

Imprint

Cover image: www.ingimage.com

This book is a translation from the original published under ISBN 978-3-330-76611-2.

Publisher:
Sciencia Scripts
is a trademark of
Dodo Books Indian Ocean Ltd. and OmniScriptum S.R.L publishing group

120 High Road, East Finchley, London, N2 9ED, United Kingdom
Str. Armeneasca 28/1, office 1, Chisinau MD-2012, Republic of Moldova, Europe
Managing Directors: Ieva Konstantinova, Victoria Ursu
info@omniscriptum.com

Printed at: see last page
ISBN: 978-620-8-53623-7

Dedication

To my parents, Cirino Marques da *Rocha (in memorí) and Quitéria de Barros da Rocha, for the dedication with which they raised their children, with honesty, dignity and simplicity.*

To my son, Erick da Rocha Dake, a gift from God, the joy of my life.

To my husband, Samuel Granato Hoelz, for his dedication, affection and support.

Special Thanks

To Professor Luciana Patrícia Fernandes Abbade, my dear supervisor, for welcoming me, for her friendship, affection, patience, persistence and determination; for her infinite understanding in difficult times, for taking my hand and guiding me along this path. Without you, none of this would have been possible. I cannot express my gratitude enough. Thank you so much.

Thank you

To GOD, for all the graces I have received, for giving me the strength to overcome difficulties, for the right paths at uncertain times, for another stage in my life.

I would like to thank Professor Valéria de Castilho Palhares for her affection, dedication, competence and availability as co-supervisor. Your support was fundamental.

To Professor Hélio Amante Miot, for his exquisite statistical work. His participation was decisive.

To Professor Márcia Aparecida Nuevo Gatti, for her generosity, for believing in me and contributing to my professional growth, my deepest gratitude. To Professor *Magda Cristina Queiroz DellAqua, for her warm welcome, sympathy, debate of ideas and encouragement of critical thinking. It's an honour to have you as members of the panel, you are an example to be followed. I am deeply grateful for your contributions and suggestions, which were so important and enriching.*

To the professionals at the Centre for Distance Education and Information Technologies in Health (NEAD.TIS) at the Botucatu Medical School - Unesp: Denise de Cássia Moreira Zonoff, Ana Silvia Sartori Barraviera Seabra Ferreira and Lucas Frederico Arantes, for welcoming us so well, helping us and promptly participating in this work, as well as contributing immensely to the development of the thematic short course.

To Taís Lopes Saranholi, who contributed immensely to the completion of this research, especially in carrying out the questionnaires, tabulating and typing the data and preparing the thematic short course. It was a pleasure to have you by my side on this journey.

To Raquel Colenci and Taynara Valério Santos for their contribution to this work, especially in preparing the thematic short course and the video lessons.

To the teaching staff of the Professional Master's Degree in Nursing - Postgraduate Programme in

Nursing of *the Nursing* Department of *the Botucatu Medical School - UNESP, I would like to thank you for the opportunity and privilege of being able to study for a Master's Degree, which has contributed to my professional and scientific training.*

To dear Manuela Botari de Mello Braga (Manú), thank you so much for your encouragement and for the attention you always paid to all of us when you were secretary of the Postgraduate Nursing programme. And to César Eduardo Guimarães for his patience in helping me, at so many moments, with my bureaucratic difficulties during the Postgraduate Programme in Nursing.

To all the teachers on the Nursing Assistant course at SENAC Bauru, where I took my first steps in nursing. And to the professors of the undergraduate nursing programme at the Sacred Heart University, for their conviviality and learning.

To my fellow nurses from the Municipal Health Department of Bauru, the ILSL, SORRI and FAMESP for their collaboration and willingness to take part in the research, even though they were overwhelmed by work.

To my dear friends at the Mary Dota Health Unit for their affection, friendship, presence and support, for being, without a doubt, part of my life.

To the nurses of the Nursing Division of the Lauro de Souza Lima Institute, for my absences during this period.

My Master's colleagues, the nurses: Drieli da Silva Valente, Lilian Salgado Cunha, Luciana Mendes Amadeu and especially Elda Garbo Pinto for her encouragement. We laughed, cried and helped each other; we shared moments of learning, it was a unique experience.

My dear friends, Terezinha Aparecida Rodrigues de Araújo, Adriana and Cristina Lopes Ferreira da Rocha, Cleide Hipólito da Silva, Luana Ribeiro Garcia Marzagão, Eliete Alves and Shirleyde Andrade Né. Always there, no matter the distance.

To *my father Cirino Marques da Rocha (ín memorían) for the values he taught me and his unconditional love. Especially to my mother, Quitéria de Barros da Rocha, for teaching me the value of study, encouraging me to read from an early age and, above all, for giving up her dreams so that we, her children, could realise ours.*

To my beloved son, Erick da Rocha Dake, for his tenderness, for his very existence that gives me the courage to live. Forgive me for being absent from so many moments of your life, being your mum is a learning experience.

To Samuel Granato Hoelz, my beloved husband, for his presence in my life, for his trust, dedication and patient waiting in *times of absence.* "Who *will ever say that there is reason in things done by the heart? And who will say that there is no reason?" (Renato Russo).*

To my siblings, Cláudia Aparecida Marques da Rocha and João Batista Marques da Rocha, for their constant support. To my dear nieces, Beatriz da Rocha Neves and Tayná da Rocha Oliveira, for their affection. And my beloved little nephews, Pedro Henrique and Miguel, who brighten up our family.

To my mother-in-law, Ana Margarida Granato, who took me in like a daughter. And my aunt, Edmea Aparecida de Barros Feige, for her affection, care and dedication to me. And my godmother and aunt, Luzia Marques Fernandes (ín memoriam), who always encouraged me and was proud of me.

Finally, my sincere thanks go to all those who contributed in one way or another so that this journey could be completed.

Epigraph

"There's nothing we have complete ***control over*** except our ***thoughts"***

René Descartes (1596-1650)

SUMMARY

Introduction: Skin wounds are a serious public health and nursing care problem. There are few studies evaluating nurses' knowledge of wound care. **Objectives: To** identify nurses' knowledge about caring for patients with wounds treated in the public health care network**.** To identify the knowledge and clinical practice of nurses working in the public healthcare network. **Method:** A cross-sectional, descriptive and analytical study with 166 nurses working in public healthcare institutions in the municipality of Bauru, who answered a structured questionnaire between May and September 2014, prepared by two specialists, and the answers considered appropriate according to systematic reviews and guidelines. Categorical variables were represented by percentage fractions and compared between subgroups using the chi-square test. These were compared using generalised linear models. The product proposed was the development of a short thematic course in a virtual environment for training in the area of wounds. **Results:** Predominance of females (88%), mean age 37.2 years; 10.7 years of undergraduate study and 9.9 years in post. The majority were graduates of private educational institutions. The predominant place of work was in the hospital network (41.6%), with a predominance of care roles (85.5%). Training during graduation was considered good by 78%, and 64.5% reported that they updated themselves in some way

about wounds. In addition, 86.3% of the nurses stated that they treat patients with wounds and 62.7% that there are dressing protocols in their institution; 65.1% answered that the nurse carries out a nursing consultation and prescribes standardised dressings; and that the dressing is carried out by the nursing assistant/technician (91.6%). According to 74.7%, the professional who carries out the dressing follows the nurse's prescription. Among therapeutic methods, collagenase ointment is the most widely known (96.4%) and used (78.9%). The unna boot is known by 80.1 per cent, but used by 16.3 per cent; and negative pressure therapy is used by only 1.8 per cent of professionals. As for specific cognitive knowledge of wounds, the median score was 5.6, with 58.4 per cent having a good score and 26.7 per cent a fair score. The highest median percentage of correct answers, 79%, was in neuropathic ulcers; and the lowest in clinical assessment (general assessment of the wound and concepts of colonisation and infection), with a median of 42%, with a statistically significant difference (**p<0**.05). There was no association between the number of correct answers and the time or institution of graduation, training on wounds during graduation, professional updating, wound care and the role performed. However, nurses who performed dressings had a better score for pressure ulcers; and those who updated their training had a better score for venous and arterial ulcers. Those who carried out nursing consultations and prescribed dressings scored better in cleaning, antisepsis and debridement. **Conclusion:** The study was able to detect deficiencies mainly in the knowledge of the concepts of critical colonisation and infection, and of some recommended practices for wound care, such as: lack of protocols and failure to treat venous ulcers with compression. This highlighted the need to **develop an "Update on wounds and dressings" course in a virtual environment.**

Key words: nurses, nursing, skin ulcers, dressings, nursing care, education.

SUMMARY

CHAPTER 1

PRESENTATION

Since I was a child, university was a dream and, over time, it became a commitment. In search of professional qualifications and better working conditions, I found nursing. I studied nursing assistant at Senac in Bauru and quickly found a place in the labour market.

My desire to learn and know more led me to study for a degree in Nursing and Obstetrics, which I completed in 2006 at the Sacred Heart University (USC). Whilst still an undergraduate, I passed the public examination for the Bauru Municipal Health Department (SMS) and the Lauro de Souza Lima Bauru Institute (ILSL) of the State Health Department (SES/SP).

After an arduous career, I worked two jobs, when I left in the morning I left my six-year-old son sleeping, and when I returned it was night and he was asleep again. The experience of being born into a humble family, having an early pregnancy, family and financial difficulties gave me maturity. In this way, I try to reflect on life's opportunities, overcoming obstacles, barriers and social determinism.

In these 17 years in nursing, the last nine of which as a nurse, I've had the opportunity to work in Basic Health Units, Municipal Reference Units and Urgency and Emergency Units. As well as constantly taking part in events, courses, congresses, seminars, symposiums, workshops, meetings and conferences, I've also studied some specialisations.

During my undergraduate nursing degree, Prof Dr Maria Helena Borgato instilled in us a restlessness for research. As time went by, I dreamed of studying for a master's degree, so I started studying English, as I needed a better qualification and instrumentalisation to work professionally.

In the second year of the course, in 2002, together with Nurse Ana Amélia da Silva Escobar, I began a research project entitled **"The repercussions of leprosy in the family context: the patient's perception", under the guidance of** Nurse Noemi Garcia de Almeida Galan.

I even got financial help from the ILSL to travel and present my first paper at the 16th International Leprosy Congress in Salvador-BA. I presented my second piece of research in 2005, **entitled "Nursing Care in the Surgical Centre: The Patient's View", under the guidance of Prof.** Márcia Regina Alves Rocha, at the 66th Nursing Week of the Universidade Sagrado Coração, during a regular internship, in partnership with Nurse Nilde Queiroz de Almeida Lima, at the time head of the Surgical Centre at the Hospital Beneficência Portuguesa.

As my Course Conclusion Paper (TCC), back in 2005, together with my friends, Eliete Alves and Rita de Cássia Silva, I carried out the research: **"The professional influence on the quality of life and health in employees of a penitentiary in the state of São Paulo",** under the guidance of

Professor Maria Helena Borgato. At the time, the Capstone didn't meet the same standards as it does today, so I didn't worry about presenting and publishing the research.

I started my first specialisation in Public Health with an emphasis on the ESF in my final year of undergraduate studies (2006), also at USC. My monograph was entitled **"Evaluation of vaccination coverage in the campaign against poliomyelitis in the municipality of Bauru, between 2004 and 2010"**, under the guidance of my dear Professor Solange Nardo Marques Cardoso.

In 2008 I took a specialisation course in Urgency and Emergency Nursing at ESAP (Londrina) and wrote a monograph in partnership with fellow nurses Ana Rosa Viaro Jardim and Gislene Aparecida Garcia Kimura, **entitled "External causes of** mortality in the municipality of Bauru, between **2004 and 2007"**, under the guidance of Professor Maria José Sanches Marin. I presented this work at the VII Biennial Nursing Conference at the Botucatu Medical School (FMB), Unesp, in 2011.

I also took a specialisation course in Health Management at the Open University of Brazil/FMB, Unesp, in 2010. I wrote the paper **"Vaccination coverage and its effectiveness: a review of the literature"**, under the guidance of Professor Cláudia Helena Bronzatto Luppi.

In 2014, I presented a paper entitled **"Evidence on the efficacy and** effectiveness of vaccines: a review", at the 1st São Paulo Congress of COREN SP, in São Paulo; and an abstract of my master's dissertation**, entitled "Knowledge** and practice of nurses on caring for patients **with wounds"**, at the 5th Brazilian Congress of Nursing in Dermatology, in Búzios, Rio de Janeiro.

It's been a long road, from the selection process and approval to completing my Master's degree. In the first half of 2011, I started as a special student on the Professional Master's Degree in Nursing at the Postgraduate Programme in Nursing, Department of Nursing, Botucatu Medical School - Unesp. In 2013, I was approved as a regular student and began the **research** project "Evaluation of the knowledge of nurses in the health care network in the municipality of Bauru (SP) about caring for patients with wounds: ªcross-sectional study", **under the guidance of the** esteemed Prof Dr Luciana Patrícia Fernandes Abbade and co-supervision of Prof Dr Valéria de Castilho Palhares.

I began my formal supervision and participation in specialisation course examinations. I began supervising monographs and exam boards (Workers' Health and Human Ecology) at the Sergio Arouca National School of Public Health/Fiocruz for Karina Fuzisaka Ferreira - Health service waste management and its relevance to workers' health. 2013 and Denise Vitorio - Social service and workers' health. 2013. After monograph orientation (Specialisation in Nursing in Surgical Centres) - Passo 1/UNIASSELVI by Flávio Antônio Sampaio - Accidents at work involving sharps among nursing workers. 2014.

Since I began my professional activities, over the years I have come to reflect on the peculiarities of wound treatment and the commitment I have to develop care actions for these patients at the ILSL as well as in primary care.

Professional experience has shown that the implementation of rules and routines for the proper care of patients with wounds brings several benefits, such as a reduction in the cost of treatment, short-term improvements and fewer dressing changes. Faced with these questions, we drew up a questionnaire (Appendix A) with the aim of checking some aspects that may be related to nurses' knowledge of dressings.

CHAPTER 2

INTRODUCTION

2.1 The role of nurses in caring for people with skin wounds

Care for people with skin wounds should be multi-professional, involving doctors, nurses, occupational therapists, physiotherapists and nutritionists, psychologists and biologists, among others. However, in daily practice, wound care at the different levels of health services is the responsibility of nurses and requires appropriate qualifications from them.[1] This care is not just limited to performing dressings, characterised solely by a technical task in compliance with medical prescriptions.

Nurses play a fundamental role in the prevention, assessment and treatment of wounds, requiring technical and scientific knowledge. With the development of nursing, characterised by more technical and specialised work, nurses have become a more prominent member of the multidisciplinary team, especially in the care of patients with skin wounds. Advances in treatment methods in this area have made nursing aware of the need for updating and better technical and scientific training.

The autonomy of nurses in the treatment of skin wounds is highlighted when they develop specific competence and specialised action, with the opportunity to make decisions that are dependent, interdependent and independent of the medical and multi-professional team. Obviously, this autonomy is linked to knowledge and recognition of their limitations and, consequently, to their clinical competence, which will be full with the application of the Systematisation of Nursing Care.[2]

According to the code of ethics for nursing professionals[7], nurses are responsible for carrying out activities inherent to caring for individuals and the community, in order to promote actions that provide well-being. Among the nurses' duties, it can be seen that, in relation to the treatment of skin lesions, the professional, as the executor or supervisor of care, relies on knowledge obtained during their training and during their search for updating.[1]

Nurses need to have adequate knowledge so that their work can be comprehensive and satisfactory, in order to provide the best care for those suffering from these conditions. To do this, they must know the anatomy and physiology of the skin, the physiology of healing, the factors that interfere with the healing process, the main causes of wounds and the resources available for treatment. All this knowledge, together with skills and attitudes, must be backed up by the Professional Practice Act, which validates their actions and supports their autonomy. In light of these issues, the importance of the nurse's role is highlighted, whether as a carer or educator, in the prevention and treatment of skin wounds.[3]

As already mentioned, nursing professionals play an important role in wound care. Careful and attentive clinical assessment will result in excellent care and successful nursing work.

The importance of applying the nursing process to patient care is emphasised, guaranteeing a comprehensive approach by identifying the needs presented and the quality of care. By means of attitudes, methods and techniques for prevention, protection, promotion and rehabilitation, nurses seek to balance a healthy condition for human beings by planning, organising and carrying out their work, basing it on the problematisation arising from the relationship between health and illness.

The nursing process is a scientific method for carrying out professional practice systematically and demonstrably more effectively. It consists of a fundamental instrument that provides organisation and direction to nursing activities for the Systematisation of Nursing Care (SNC), under the responsibility of the nurse. **It is** driven by the need for a **"critical, reflective and scientifically based" care process,** consisting of data collection, diagnosis, planning, implementation of actions and evaluation of the results.[4,5]

The Curriculum Guidelines of the National Education Council (CNE) define the principles, foundations, conditions and procedures in educational training that should be considered by the institutions of the Brazilian education system, with specifications for each teaching area.[6]

The specific competences and skills required for the training of nurses, as expressed in the Curriculum Guidelines, reveal some aspects that support the exercise of quality care, which is expected for their professional practice.[6]

Efforts by training institutions to articulate this methodological reference with the construction of the competences of knowing, doing and being in the profession are essential. It should be emphasised **that the use of the term "competences" in** Resolution No. 03/2001 CNE/SES reflects the ability to do (professional practice) based on the necessary knowledge (know-how), which together enables nurses to act with competence, now understood as a set of good quality knowledge and practice.[3]

According to COFEN Decree No. 94.406/87 (2014), Article 8 describes the **role of nurses in relation to wound care, stating that: "It is** the nurse's role to carry out nursing care of greater technical complexity and requiring scientifically based knowledge and the ability to make **immediate decisions", showing the importance of the nurse's role** in caring for people with skin wounds.[7]

There are various materials and methods for treating skin wounds. In order to provide the best care for each patient, there is a need for assessment and treatment protocols to unify and contribute to more practical and qualified care. The creation of a protocol can be guided by demands and objectives linked to the interests of a professional group, a multi-professional team, the institution or even those originating from all these groups. However, the protocol cannot be dissociated from the overarching objective, which is quality of care.[8] Protocols also help the autonomy of the nursing professional, by guaranteeing legal, technical and scientific backing.[2]

Professionals must be familiar with the materials used to ensure they are used correctly, and constantly re-evaluate whether the products should be changed or remain on the wounds. This requires continuing education to keep their knowledge and practices up to date, providing specific and differentiated care and contributing to improving the quality of life of people with skin wounds.

In a recent integrative review on the role of nurses in wound care, Dutton et al[9] concluded that there is little consensus on the level of competence, educational requirements and qualifications needed for nurses to provide wound care. However, there was some evidence that nurse care of wounds reduces healing time and the prevalence of pressure ulcers.

Some studies have assessed the level of knowledge of nursing professionals related to wounds. According to Ferreira et al (2014)[10], nurses' knowledge and evidence-based practice begins during their undergraduate studies. This knowledge is a determining factor in future prevention and treatment of patients with wounds under their responsibility, along with other health professionals.

2.2 Definition and classification of skin wounds

A wound occurs when there is discontinuity of epithelial tissue, mucous membranes or organs with damage to their basic functions, as a result of a chemical, physical or microbial agent. A cutaneous wound is characterised by an injury with loss of tissue, affecting the epidermis, dermis and sometimes reaching the subcutaneous cellular tissue or deeper tissues.[11]

Skin wounds should be assessed in terms of etiology, location, size, type, stage, degree of contamination, characteristics of the bed, edge, exudate, odour and the condition of the surrounding skin. A clinical assessment of the patient and other factors that influence the healing process is also necessary.[12] To facilitate clinical assessment, skin wounds can be classified in terms of their origin, depth, complexity, healing time and form, and bacterial load.[13]

In terms of origin or cause, they can be: traumatic - caused accidentally by mechanical agents (cuts, punctures), chemical and physical agents (heat, cold, radiation); surgical - caused intentionally by sharp surgical instruments. Originated by underlying diseases, such as venous, arterial, neuropathic and others.[14]

Depending on their depth, they can be: superficial or partial - when they only affect the epidermis and part of the dermis; and deep or total - when in addition to the upper layers they affect the subcutaneous tissue, muscles and bones.[11]

In terms of complexity, acute cutaneous wounds can be simple or complex. The former occur in surgical incisions that are sutured and have no complications during tissue repair. The latter, on the other hand, occur when there are systemic or local complications related to the patient's general condition and the technical-surgical procedure adopted. The main complications that make a surgical wound complex are: haematoma, seroma, soft tissue infections and dehiscence.[15]

In terms of healing time, wounds are classified as acute or chronic. Acute wounds are those caused by surgery or trauma, in which repair usually takes place within the expected timeframe, without difficulties or complications. Chronic wounds, on the other hand, are those that do not heal in the expected time and are susceptible to complications. Examples of the latter are venous ulcers, arterial ulcers, neuropathic ulcers and pressure ulcers.[11]

Skin wounds can heal by first, second or third intention. The first occurs when an acute wound is allowed to heal after approximating its edges (direct suturing of the edges, graft or flap). Healing by second intention occurs when a wound is allowed to heal by itself. Third intention healing, on the other hand, occurs when a wound is surgically corrected after the formation of granulation tissue, in order to provide better functional and aesthetic results.[16]

In terms of bacterial load, acute traumatic wounds are classified as follows:[17]

> Clean: no microorganisms;
>
> Clean-contaminated: injury less than 6 hours between trauma and care, without significant contamination;
>
> Contaminated: injuries sustained over 6 hours (trauma and care), with no sign of infection;
>
> Infected: presence of an infectious agent at the site, and a lesion with evidence of an intense inflammatory reaction and tissue destruction, with the possible presence of purulent secretion.

For chronic wounds, the classification in terms of bacterial load is different and goes as follows:[18]

> Contaminated: non-replicating bacteria in the wound bed;
>
> Colonisation: replicating bacteria in the wound bed, but with insufficient pathogenicity and number to inhibit the normal healing process. Colonisation is also characterised by a lack of host immune response;
>
> Critical colonisation: presence of replicating bacteria in the tissue, now in greater numbers (bioburden) and with pathogenicity capable of inhibiting the healing process. Colonised wounds do not have good granulation tissue and may have a yellowish, greenish (when colonised by pseudomonas) or wine-coloured bottom. In addition, they have excessive exudation and a foul odour.[4, 5] Systemic antibiotics are not indicated, as they have not been shown to improve ulcer healing, and local wound care is more indicated.[6]
>
> Infection: penetration and proliferation of bacteria deep into the tissues around the ulcer leading to erysipelas, cellulitis or bacterial lymphangitis. Treatment with systemic antibiotics is necessary.

There is also a classification for skin wounds based on the colours of the wound bed using the RYB System (**Red, Yellow, Black**). The wound is categorised by observing the red, yellow or black colours and their variations. There are also classifications based on the appearance of the exudate or the size of the wound.[13]

As mentioned above, the various forms of classification help clinical assessment and, consequently, favour the most appropriate therapeutic approach, according to the local conditions of the wound.

2.3 Epidemiology and cost of treating the main skin wounds

Among the various types of skin wounds, chronic wounds are the most prevalent in health services at all levels. The main chronic wounds are venous, arterial, pressure and neuropathic ulcers. They are usually long-lasting and have a variable therapeutic response[19].

Venous wounds are caused by chronic venous disease, with primary varicose veins and late effects of deep vein thrombosis being the main causes. It is associated with dysfunction of the calf muscle pump, which leads to chronic venous hypertension.[20] They are highly prevalent, accounting for 70% to 90% of lesions located in the lower limbs, and their common denominator is chronic venous insufficiency.[21] In Brazil, Maffei et al. carried out a study of 1755 people over the age of 15 and found a prevalence of 6.3% of active and/or healed venous ulcers, of which 2.3% occurred in men and 4% in women.[22] It is estimated that in the United States approximately 500,000 people have venous ulcers.[23]

Arterial ulcers occur due to peripheral arterial disease, which is the main manifestation of systemic atherosclerosis. They account for 10% to 25% of cases of chronic ulcers of the lower limbs.[21] The prevalence of peripheral arterial disease in the population is approximately 12%, and it affects men and women equally.[24]

Pressure ulcers are also very prevalent and are the result of prolonged pressure, especially in areas of bony prominences.[25] Pressure ulcers occur in approximately 1.5 to 3 million people in the United States.[25] In most cases, the ulcer develops in a hospital environment[26]. In a study conducted in a Brazilian university hospital, the incidence of pressure ulcers was 39.8%, varying according to the hospital unit studied, with 41.0% in the intensive care unit.[27] In another Brazilian study,[28] pressure ulcers occurred in 35.2% of patients admitted to the intensive care unit. The incidence is higher in elderly patients, patients in a coma or with neurological disorders (mainly paraplegics and tetraplegics).

Neuropathic ulcers are common in diseases that affect the peripheral nervous system, such as leprosy, alcoholism and Diabetes Mellitus, which are endemic in Brazil.[29,30,31] There are many causes and types of peripheral neuropathies, but those that lead to sensory loss and trophic changes due to denervation are responsible for the greatest risk of foot ulcers. Due to the high prevalence of neuropathic ulcers, there are manuals from the Ministry of Health, in association with other health management bodies, which give special focus to these ulcers.

Some studies show that between 4.8% and 7% of diabetic patients have or have had foot ulcers; 1.4% have had amputations and 67% had one or more risk factors for amputation. There are approximately 20 million diabetic patients in the United States, and 10% to 15% of these patients are at risk of developing foot ulcers at some point during their lives. Foot ulcers represent the most common cause of hospitalisation for diabetic patients in Western countries [29,32].

Chronic skin wounds, due to their high prevalence, difficulty in healing and high recurrence rates, cause a high socio-economic impact related to costs to the health and social security system, in terms of professional care, use of therapeutic resources for healing, absenteeism from work and reduced quality of life, which involves daily and leisure activities.[33,34]

The costs of treating wounds have been high and increase even more when there is no established standard of care and no trained professionals to carry it out. In general, evidence-based practice has not yet been incorporated by the majority of health professionals who are responsible for wound care.

The financial cost of this problem is the subject of several studies. Some studies have looked at the cost of treating the main causes of chronic ulcers, such as venous, pressure and neuropathic ulcers.

In the United States, the annual cost of treating venous ulcers is estimated to be between 1.9 and 2.5 billion dollars[35], while in the United Kingdom 1.3 per cent of the health budget is spent on treating venous ulcers.[36] Also in the United States, the annual cost of treating pressure ulcers has been estimated at 5 billion dollars a year.[37]

In Sweden, a study suggested that the cost of a single episode of foot ulcer was 7,850 dollars if amputation was avoided. However, the cost rises to 52,920 dollars if amputation is necessary.[38] In the United States, an estimated 500 million dollars is spent on amputation due to foot ulcers in diabetic patients every year.[39]

There is a lack of similar data recorded in Brazil.

2.4 Therapeutic approach to chronic skin wounds

When faced with a patient with a skin wound, the therapeutic approach should initially be aimed at the cause that caused it and the patient's general condition. At the same time, local treatment of the wound should be carried out.

2.4.1 Cause-orientated approach

2.4.1.1 Venous ulcer

A number of strategies must be implemented to reduce chronic venous hypertension and its repercussions on the macrocirculation and microcirculation.[40] One of the main measures to achieve these goals is the choice of compressive therapy. Compressive therapies are mainly represented by the Unna boot, compressible elastic bands and multilayer compressive treatment.[41,42] All of these compressive methods are contraindicated if the patient has severe peripheral arterial disease, i.e. nonpalpable distal pulses or an ankle-arm index of less than 0.5.

Another measure that acts on the cause of venous ulcers is proper rest, as this reduces the effects of venous hypertension. This rest should be carried out with the lower limb elevated above the level of the heart, for 30 minutes, around three to four times during the day and throughout the night. The ideal elevation is 15 to 20 cm from the foot of the bed. This measure should not be carried out in cases where it is associated with arterial disease [43].

Surgical treatment of the venous abnormality, when possible, should be considered with the aim of eliminating or reducing the transmission of high venous pressure to the ulcerated areas[44].

2.4.1.2 Arterial ulcer

Patients with arterial ulcers should be assessed by vascular surgeons, with the aim of restoring adequate arterial flow, and may benefit from angioplasty or bypass surgery. Additional therapies include adequate pain control and keeping the limb warm.[24]

2.4.1.3 Neuropathic ulcer

For patients with neuropathies, the best measure is ulcer prevention. They should be given special advice about their shoes and have their feet systematically inspected. It is important to reduce high plantar pressure with insoles that distribute weight in the plantar region.[45]

Orthopaedic devices are used because they allow walking and reduce pressure on ulcerated and calloused areas. Specially made and customised footwear is indicated in cases of greater foot deformities, as it allows for greater width and depth. Other forms of plantar reduction or unloading include crutches, walkers and even total deprivation of contact. Guidance on weight loss is essential for overweight and obese patients.[45]

2.4.1.4 Pressure ulcers

When thinking about the approach to the cause of pressure ulcers, we have to consider that the main aetiological factors involved in their development are pressure, friction, traction forces and humidity. Prolonged pressure, especially on bony prominences, compromises microcirculation and, consequently, oxygenation of adjacent tissues. Friction of the skin against other surfaces can occur due to muscle spasticity, inadequate mobilisation of the patient or untimely removal of dressings. Damage to the stratum corneum compromises the skin's barrier function, favouring ulceration. Traction forces occur when the body moves over the skin fixed to the external surface, and there is a risk of this when the headboard is above 30°. Moisture from perspiration and prolonged contact with faeces and urine causes maceration of the skin, leading to continuity lesions that can develop into ulcers [37].

The most important therapeutic measure is to reduce or eliminate the triggering factors mentioned above. Pressure relief in ulcerated areas or those at risk of ulceration can be achieved with frequent changes of **position, water and air mattresses, pillows and some adaptable foams.** When the patient is in the lateral decubitus position, this should be around 30°, to reduce pressure on the trochanteric region.[46]

The head of the bed should always be lower than 30° to reduce traction on the sacrococcygeal area. Foam cushions or wedges are recommended to avoid direct contact between bone surfaces, especially between the knees, and cushions on the back of the leg to elevate the heels. Protection with gloves containing **water, donut cushions or rings is** not recommended**.** Sheets should always be dry, free of creases and food debris.[46]

Friction must be avoided and care must be taken when transferring patients. Dragging the patient is not recommended. We recommend using lifting devices, bearings or transfer sheets.

General skin care is important, such as keeping it clean and dry, using a gentle cleansing agent, avoiding hot water and friction, using a barrier emollient/hydrating agent and not massaging it over bony prominences. It is also essential to control bladder and bowel emptying. When this is not possible, immediate cleaning after evacuation, application of barrier moisturisers and highly absorbent nappies are necessary. The need for nutritional support should also be assessed.

2.4.2 Local wound treatment

Wound bed preparation refers to an approach that allows the clinician to systematically focus on all the critical components that hinder the healing of chronic skin wounds, in order to identify the cause of the problem and implement a programme to optimise the healing process.

To help with the implementation of the wound bed preparation concept, a group of wound care specialists created a mnemonic rule using the acronym TIME.[47]. To facilitate this assessment, the letter T refers to tissue, i.e. assessment of the presence of devitalised or non-viable tissue in the ulcer bed. The letter I refers to the presence of infection or colonisation. The letter M refers to **"moisture imbalance";** and the letter E refers to "edge"**.**

2.4.2.1 Cleaning the wound

Only saline solution or drinking water should be used to clean the wound, as various antiseptic substances (chlorhexidine, povidone-iodine, acetic acid, sodium hypochlorite, potassium permanganate, among others) are cytotoxic and can delay healing.[48]

2.4.2.2 Approach to devitalised tissues (TIME letter "T")

In the presence of non-viable tissues, debridement is necessary because these tissues, as well as favouring infection, do not allow the formation of good granulation tissue and adequate re-epithelialisation.[49]

There are basically five forms of debridement: autolytic, chemical, mechanical, surgical and biological. Autolytic debridement can be achieved with occlusive dressings, through the action of enzymes in the exudate that remains in contact with the ulcer. Examples of these dressings are hydrogels and hydrocolloids. Chemical debridement is carried out by applying various enzymes, including collagenase and papain. However, there is no evidence of its effectiveness in randomised controlled studies.[50,51] Mechanical debridement can be carried out using surgical instruments or by applying dressings, which vary from wet to dry. The main disadvantage of this technique is that it is non-selective, removing viable tissue along with devitalised tissue. Negative pressure therapy (e.g. V.A.C®) is an alternative, and its use has increased in recent years.[52]

2.4.2.3 Approach to infection/colonisation of the ulcer bed (TIME letter I)

In chronic ulcers, bacteria can form complex structures called biofilms. Biofilms are communities of microorganisms surrounded by an extracellular polysaccharide matrix. Bacteria with biofilms are better protected and more resistant to the body's defences, antiseptics and both topical and systemic antibiotics.[53]

Controlling critical colonisation in chronic ulcers plays a vital role in the healing process. The local approach to ulcers with critical colonisation can be surgical or chemical debridement. Surgical debridement is the quickest way to reduce the bacterial load, but it is a non-selective method and can be painful. Occlusive dressings with silver are options that control excess exudation and promote a reduction in the bacterial load.[54]

Examples include activated charcoal with silver, hydrofibre with silver and alginate with calcium. These dressings can be changed according to saturation, every 3 to 7 days.[54] It is worth emphasising that systemic antibiotics are not indicated as they are unable to act on these biofilm-forming bacteria.

Soft tissue infections manifest clinically with erythema, oedema, pain and local heat in the tissues around the wound. Fever, tachycardia, hypotension and leucocytosis may accompany the condition. It is important to carry out blood cultures in cases with systemic repercussions and treatment should be carried out with systemic antibiotics and, where possible, debridement of the infected tissues.

2.4.2.4 Keeping the environment moist (letter M in TIME)

The amount of exudate in the ulcer should also be assessed, ideally keeping the bed moist. Excessive exudate must be combated because, as well as favouring infection, it brings discomfort to the patient. On the other hand, dehydration of the ulcer bed should be avoided and combated, as it favours the formation of devitalised tissues.[48]

Therefore, in order to provide an optimal environment for healing, there are a number of occlusive dressings that can be indicated according to the characteristics of the wounds. For wounds with excessive exudation, alginate, charcoal with silver, charcoal and alginate, hydropolymer and hydrofibre dressings are indicated. For wounds with a mild to moderate amount of exudation, hydrocolloid dressings and hydrogels are indicated.[(48)]

2.4.2.5 Wound edge assessment (TIME letter E)

The systematic and structured assessment of the wound bed includes the evaluation of the wound edge and periulcer tissues. Detached and undermined edges indicate poor evolution of the healing process. Indications of good evolution are when the edges are glued and at the same level as the wound bed.

The edges may also be hyperkeratotic, especially in dry wounds. It is important to gently remove the hyperkeratosis and use dressings to improve hydration, in order to favour keratinocyte migration. Macerated edges also hinder keratinocyte migration. They are usually associated with excessive exudation or the use of dressings that cause hyperhydration or do not absorb the exudate. In this case, dressings that absorb excess exudate are essential.

The periulcer tissues can present contact eczema and this also hinders wound healing. The lesions are usually pruritic and secondary to the sensitisation that patients develop over time, especially to topical antibiotics (neomycin, sulfa, gentamicin, among others), lanolin and antiseptics (povidone-iodine).[55]

2.5 Justification

Despite the social importance and direct responsibility of nurses in caring for people with skin wounds, there are few systematised studies evaluating the practice and knowledge of this professional in relation to this care.

Some studies show a lack of knowledge among undergraduate nursing students, due to flaws in the teaching method and insufficient workload for learning about wound care during the undergraduate course.[56,57] Other studies expose the lack of specialisation, organisation and updating of professionals who have already graduated and are active in the job market.[10] Others show that the lack of records and communication means that the wound is cared for at different stages and by different professionals, in an inappropriate way, due to the lack of protocols and systematised assessment.[58]

2.6 Study question

What is the practice and knowledge of nurses about caring for people with skin wounds in public health care networks?

2.7 Study hypothesis

The hypothesis of this study is that identifying the practice and knowledge of nurses related to caring for patients with wounds will have an impact on the scientific community, as it will be possible to diagnose the role of nursing professionals in dealing with this highly prevalent health problem, making it possible to create strategies to optimise care and teaching.

CHAPTER 3

OBJECTIVES

3.1 General Objective

id To identify the knowledge and practice of nurses working in the public health care network of the municipality of Bauru on the care of patients with wounds.

3.2 Specific objectives

D To outline the sociodemographic profile of nurses;

C Characterise your professional training and updating;

D Describe the therapeutic methods known and used for wounds;

J Identify specific knowledge about skin wounds;

C Correlate nurses' knowledge with information related to professional training and practice.

E Design a thematic short course *(online)* for health professionals on updating wounds and dressings.

CHAPTER 4

METHOD

4.1 Type of Study

This is a cross-sectional, descriptive and analytical study with a quantitative approach, which meets the proposed objective of quantifying and analysing nurses' practice and knowledge of caring for patients with wounds.

4.2 Study site

The study was carried out in public healthcare institutions in the municipality of Bauru:

U Basic Health Units (UBS);

U Family Health Unit (USF);

U Urgency and Emergency Units (Emergency Care Unit - UPAS and Emergency Room);

Municipal Reference Outpatient Health Units;

Z Lauro de Souza Lima Institute;

H State Hospital Bauru;

H Hospital de Base Bauru;

H State Hospital Manoelde Abreu State Hospital in Bauru.

4.3 Population and Sample

The research participants were nurses who provide care to patients with wounds in the above-mentioned units, regardless of their length of service.

According to the National Registry of Health Establishments (CNES)[1], in 2013 there were 412 registered nurses in the municipality of Bauru, of which 166 made up the sample for this study. The professionals were located as follows: 165 at the State Hospital, 15 at the Manoel de Abreu Hospital, 83 at the Base Hospital, 25 at the Lauro de Souza Lima Institute and 124 nurses working at the Municipal Health Department, which covers the primary care network, municipal reference health units and urgent and emergency care units.

The data collection methodology was a structured questionnaire (Appendix A), applied by the researchers to a convenience sample. All nurses who were not on holiday or sick leave during data collection and who agreed to take part by signing the Informed Consent Form (ICF - Appendix B) were included in the study.

The research was approved by the scientific and ethics committees of the institutions surveyed (Annexes A, B, C, D) and by the Research Ethics Committee of the Botucatu Medical School (Annex E). When filling in the questionnaire, the participating nurses were not identified, preserving their anonymity.

4.4 Variables

Z Age;

S Sex: Male and Female;

Year and institution of graduation;

L Current place of work: Basic Health Units (UBS), Family Health Units (USF), Emergency Units (UPAS and Pronto Socorro), Municipal Reference Outpatient Health Units or Hospitals (Infirmary and Outpatient);

N Length of time working as a nurse;

T Length of time working at the institution where the research is being carried out;

A Whether or not to treat patients with wounds;

Information related to training/updating knowledge on wounds;

[1] National Register of Health Establishments -CNES. [cited http:// cnes.datasus.gov.br/. Accessed: 08 Apr 2013].

J Information on clinical practice in wounds;

Cognitive assessment of knowledge of topics related to the care of patients with wounds: 37 questions related to the subject and the survey participant ticked for each one whether they agreed, disagreed or couldn't answer (Appendix A, item 4);

E Overall score on the knowledge questionnaire: when less than 25 per cent got it right, it was considered bad, 26 to 50 per cent fair, 51 to 75 per cent good and above 75 per cent excellent;

P Percentage of correct answers per specific topic in the knowledge questionnaire: within the 37-question knowledge questionnaire (Appendix B, item 4), the questions were grouped into six main topics.

Questions related to pressure ulcers (questions 8, 14, 28, 29, 30 and 32), ulcers venous and arterial (questions 7, 10, 20, 25, 37), neuropathic ulcers (questions 9, 16, 31); clinical assessment of wounds, such as general assessment of the wound and concepts of colonisation and infection (questions 1, 2,

3, 11, 12, 13, 15, 23, 36); concepts of cleaning, antisepsis and debridement (questions 18, 19, 21, 22, 24, 27, 33, 34, 35); and dressings (questions 4, 5, 6, 17, 25).The median percentage of correct answers on each topic was calculated and compared within the subgroups.

4.5 Data Collection Instrument

The questionnaire was drawn up by two wound specialists, and the answers were considered appropriate according to a systematic review and a specific, up-to-date guideline. [40, 46,48] The data was collected using a pre-tested standard questionnaire (Appendix A), which was applied by the researchers and submitted to an evaluation by postgraduate nursing students from the Professional Master's Degree course at the Nursing Department of the Botucatu Medical School - UNESP, in order to assess its clarity and relevance. After this pre-test, some questions were reworded for better understanding.

The reliability of the questionnaire used was estimated using the Cronbach's alpha coefficient, which was 0.799.[59]

4.6 Data Collection

The nurses or managers of the unit were contacted beforehand by telephone or e-mail to arrange a date on which the researcher explained the objectives of the research and invited the nurses to take part. Those who agreed to take part signed the ICF (Appendix B). Only after signing did the participants answer a questionnaire in the presence of the researcher.

4.7 Data Analysis

Categorical variables were represented by percentage fractions and compared between subgroups using the chi-square test and analysis of residuals from the contingency table.

Quantitative variables were represented by means and standard deviations or medians and quartiles (p25-p75) if normality was not demonstrated by the Lilliefors test.

The subgroups were compared using generalised linear models appropriate to the probability distributions found.

The items in the questionnaire were assessed for their ease and ability to discriminate. Sets of items with similar behaviour were explored using cluster analysis and exploratory factor analysis after **varimax** rotation.

The total number of correct answers was assessed according to the demographic and training-related variables using generalised linear models, appropriate to the probability distributions found.

The correlation between the items and the demographic and training-related variables was explored using multidimensional scaling. Data was tabulated in MS Excel 2010 and analysed using IBM SPSS 20.0 software. A value of $p<0.05$ was considered significant.

4.8 Sample sizing

A pre-test was carried out with 100 nurses from the public health care network in the municipality of Bauru, to assess the need for sample supplementation, based on multivariate comparisons with an estimate of 5 participants for each variable included in the final model and at least 10 correct answers for each item. It was expected that up to 150 questionnaires would be needed for sample sufficiency. A total of 166 professional nurses were interviewed.

4.9 Product

Development of **the thematic** short **course "Update on** cutaneous **wounds** and **dressings"**, in a virtual environment, with the support of the Centre for Distance Education and Information Technologies in Health (NEAD.TIS) of the Botucatu Medical School - Unesp.

The target audience is healthcare professionals who deal with wound care on a daily basis, including nurses, doctors, nutritionists, nursing and medical graduates, and members of the nursing team.

Divided into five modules - Clinical assessment of wounds - general assessment of the wound **and concepts of colonisation and infection; Concepts of cleaning and debridement; Dressings; Approach to pressure, venous, arterial and neuropathic ulcers; the** course will be based on current scientific and technological knowledge, with the aim of helping health professionals who assess and care for patients in these conditions, providing support for qualified care at the different levels of care for patients with acute and chronic wounds, such as: venous ulcers, arterial ulcers, neuropathic ulcers and pressure ulcers.

The course has been registered with UNESP's Pro-Rectory for Extension (PROEX) (Annex F and G). Students who pass the assessment offered will be eligible to receive a certificate and accreditation of completion, issued by PROEX and the Virtual Medical School (EMV), linked to the Centre for Distance Education and Health Information Technology (NEAD.TIS) of the Botucatu Medical School (FMB).

The certificates issued by EMV will be backed by Unesp Resolution No. 59, of 10 July 2014, which regulates university extension courses.

taught at UNESP, and therefore validated by law.

4.10 Conflict of Interest

The authors declare no conflicts of interest.

CHAPTER 5

RESULTS

Of the total of 412 nurses, 166 (39.15%) were part of the sample, as described in Table 1. The instrument was filled in by the nurses themselves, individually, during an interview conducted by the authors, who had been duly trained by the study supervisor. Each interview lasted an average of thirty minutes. The data collected was double-entered for quality validation.

Table 1: Distribution of nurses in the public health network in the municipality of Bauru, according to institution, 2014.

Institution	Registered (n and %)	Participants (n and %)
Bauru State Hospital	165 (40,0)	53 (32,0)
Base Hospital	83 (20,0)	32 (19,0)
Lauro de Souza Lima Institute	25 (6,0)	17 (10,0)
Manoel de Abreu Hospital	15 (4,0)	5 (3,0)
Municipal Health Department	124 (30,0)	59 (36,0)
Municipal Reference Centre/Municipal Management	35 (31,0)	7 (12,0)
Basic Health Unit	33 (30,0)	25 (42,0)
Emergency Care Unit	33 (29,5)	19 (32,0)
Family Health Unit	11 (10,0)	8 (14,0)
Total	412 (100)	166 (100)

The other results will be shown in the following topics: sociodemographic profile of the population studied; professional training and updating; known/used therapeutic methods and specific knowledge about skin wounds.

Table 2 shows the results of the socio-demographic profile. Most of the participants in the survey were female, with a distribution of 88 per cent women and 12 per cent men, with a mean age of 37.2 years, 10.7 years of undergraduate study and 9.9 years of experience as a nurse.

With regard to the training institution, the following stand out: USC, with 44.6 per cent; UNIP, 19.3 per cent; Anhanguera, 12.0 per cent; Unimar, 4.8 per cent; Famema, 3.0 per cent; and Unesp, 2.4 per cent. Other public institutions totalled 3.0% and private institutions 10.8%. As for their place of work, most of the participating nurses are in the hospital network, with 41.6% working in inpatient units (wards), 9.0% in outpatient clinics and 18.1% in management. In the municipal care network, the majority of nurses work in the UBS and PSF, with 19.9% of the professionals. It should be noted that the majority of the participating nurses perform care functions (85.5%).

Table 2: Sociodemographic profile of nurses from the public health network in the municipality of Bauru, 2014.

Sociodemographic variables			
Number of professionals n (%)		166	100
Sex	Female n (%)	146	88,0
	Male n (%)	20	12,0
Age (years)	Mean (SD)	37,2	10,1
Training time	Mean (SD)	10,7	8,8
Length of Service as a Nurse	Mean (SD)	9,9	11,0
		n	%
Training institution	USC	74	44,6
	UNIP	32	19,3
	Anhanguera	20	12,0
	Unimar	8	4,8
	Famema	5	3,0
	Unesp	4	2,4
	Other Public	5	3,0
	Other Private	18	10,8
Workplace	Hospital Infirmary	69	41,6
	Basic Health Unit Family Health Unit	33	19,9
	Management Coordination	30	18,1
	Emergency Care Unit	19	11,4
	Hospital Outpatients Municipal Reference Centre	15	9,0
Role played	Assistance	142	85,5
	Administrative	24	14,5

The data on nurses' training and professional updating in relation to skin wounds is shown in Table 3. Undergraduate training was considered fair to good for 82.5 per cent of the participants. Most nurses (85.0%) reported that they always or sometimes attend to wounds. The median length of service was 5 years. One hundred and seven participants (64.5%) indicated that they keep up to date on the subject of wounds.

Table 3: Practice, training and professional updating in relation to skin wounds, of nurses from the public health network in the municipality of Bauru, 2014.

Variables on training and updating			
How did you consider the knowledge you acquired about wounds during your degree programme?		n	%
	Great	8	4,8
	Good	78	47,0
	Fair Poor	59	35,5
	Don't know Didn't answer	15	9,0
Wound care	Yes	67	40,4
	Sometimes	74	44,6
	No	25	15,1
Updates on wounds	Yes	107	64,5
	No	59	35,5
Time spent treating wounds - in years	Median	5,0	
	p25	3,0	
	p75	10,0	

Of the nine possible ways of keeping up to date in the questionnaire, the respondent could tick more than one option, with the alternatives "always", "sometimes" and "never". Considering the "always" alternative, the most frequent way of searching for information was with other nursing professionals (58.0%), followed by consulting electronic sites (40.0%) and reading scientific articles (21.0%), as shown in Graph 1.

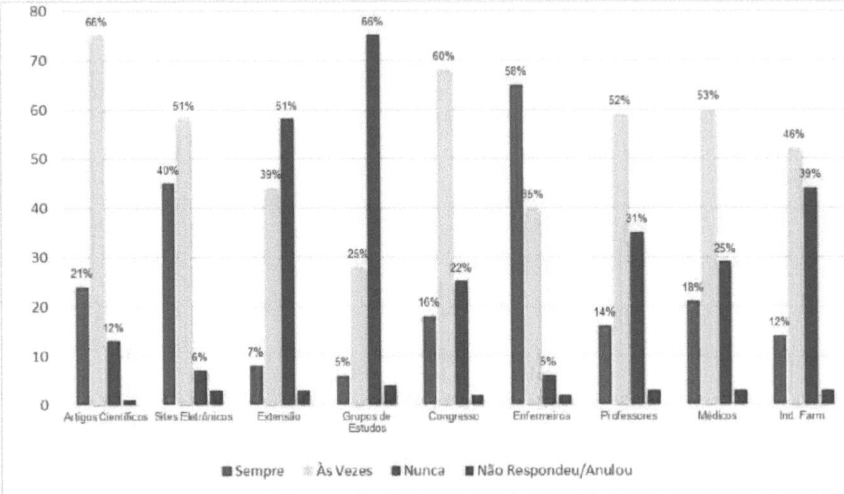

Graph 1: Resources used in professional updating - in relation to skin wounds - by nurses from the public health network in the municipality of Bauru, 2014.

After quantitatively analysing the information on clinical practice in wounds, we identified - as shown in Table 4 - that 62.7% (104) of the participants answered that there are dressing protocols in the institution. 108 nurses (65.1%) replied that the nurse carries out the nursing consultation and prescribes the standardised dressing, 152 nurses (91.6%) said that the technician/nursing assistant is the one who carries out the dressing in the institution and only nine (5.4%) replied that it is the nurse, 124 nurses (74.7%) replied that the professional who carries out the dressing follows the nurse's prescription.

While 86 nurses (51.8 per cent) replied that dressings are carried out in dressing and procedure rooms, 97 nurses (58.4 per cent) replied that medical assessment sometimes takes place when dressings are carried out or monitored, and 49 (29.5 per cent) replied that it always does, 119 participants (71.7 per cent) reported that the professional who carries out the dressing is aware of the cause of the patient's wound.

Table 4: Information on the clinical practice of nurses from the public health network in the municipality of Bauru, 2014.

Variables on clinical practice		n	%
Existence of a dressing protocol in the institution	Yes	104	62,7
	No	42	25,3
	Don't know	18	10,8
	No Answer	2	1,2

Nursing prescription/Nursing consultation/Standardised dressing	Yes	108	65,1
	No	49	29,5
	Don't know	8	4,8
	No Answer	1	0,6
Professional who performs dressings at the institution	Nursing Technician/Assistant	152	91,6
	Nurse	9	5,4
	Doctor	0	0,0
	Don't know	3	1,8
	No answer	2	1,2
Professional who prescribes the dressing	Nurse	124	74,7
	Doctor	28	16,9
	Standardised	7	4,2
	Don't know	2	1,2
	No answer	5	3,0
Where the dressings are made	Dressing/Procedure Room	86	51,8
	Bed/room/nursery	73	44,0
	No specific location	3	1,8
	Doesn't know	2	1,2
	Consultancy	1	0,6
	Others	1	0,6
	Home	0	0,0
Medical assessment - performing/monitoring dressings	Sometimes	97	58,4
	Yes	49	29,5
	No	12	7,2
	Don't know	7	4,2
	No answer	1	0,6
Know the cause of the wound	Yes	119	71,7
	Sometimes	43	25,9
	No answer	3	1,8
	No	1	0,6

With regard to the therapeutic methods for wounds known and used by nurses, it was possible to tick more than one alternative. Table 5 shows that collagenase ointment, kollagenase® or Iruxol®, is known by 160 (96.4%) and used by 131 (78.9%) professionals. Essential fatty acids (EFA) or Dersani® are known by 157 (94.6%) and used by 130 (78.3%) of the participants. Silver sulphadiazine is known by 148 (89.2%) and used by 85 (51.2%), while neomycin was mentioned by 129 (77.7%) professionals and used by 51 (30.7%). Similarly, the Unna boot is known by 133 (80.1%) professionals and used by 27 (16.3%). Negative pressure or vacuum therapy was also mentioned as being known by 42 nurses (25.3%) and used by only three (1.8%).

Table 5: Distribution of therapeutic methods known and used by nurses in the public health network in the municipality of Bauru, 2014.

Variables Therapeutic Methods	Known		Used	
	n	%	n	%
Collagenase, Kollagenase®, Iruxol®	160	96,4	131	78,9
Essential Fatty Acids (EFA), Dersani®	157	94,6	130	78,3
Sulfadiazine	148	89,2	85	51,2
Activated carbon with or without silver	146	88,0	64	38,6
Papain	144	86,7	55	33,1
Hydrocolloid	137	82,5	61	36,7
Unna boot	133	80,1	27	16,3
Neomycin, Nebacetim®	129	77,7	51	30,7
Hydrogel	120	72,3	48	28,9
Calcium alginate	113	68,1	35	21,1

Hyperbaric Oxygen Therapy	101	60,8	13	7,8
Fibrinolysin, Fibrase®	83	50,0	6	3,6
Compression elastic band	65	39,2	11	6,6
Hydrofibre with or without silver	47	28,3	9	5,4
Negative Pressure or Vacuum Therapy	42	25,3	3	1,8
None of the above	1	0,6	9	5,4
Others	7	4,2	1	0,6

Specific cognitive knowledge of wounds was measured using a 37-item questionnaire. According to the overall score achieved (Graph 2), three nurses (1.9 per cent) had a poor score, 45 (26.7 per cent) a fair score, 104 (58.4 per cent) a good score and 14 (13 per cent) an excellent score.

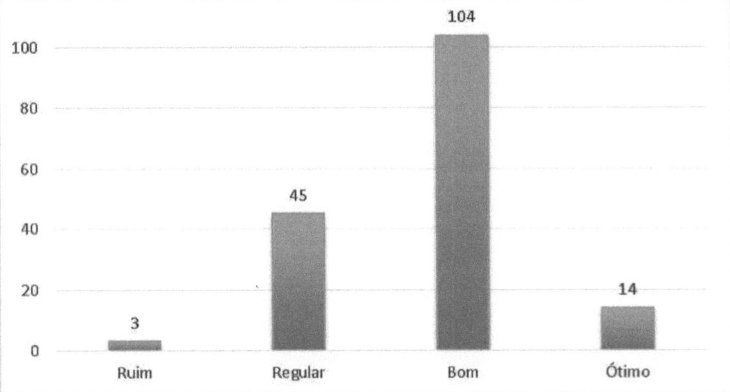

Graph 2: Score of correct answers by nurses from the public health network in the municipality of Bauru, in the questionnaire on knowledge of skin wounds, 2014.

The median score was 5.6 (from zero to 10), the 25th percentile was 4.8 and the 75th percentile was 6.7. We emphasise that 115 participants (71.4%) got more than 50% of the questions right. We would emphasise that 50% of the questions achieved 61.5% correct answers (median). The most difficult questions had up to 41% correct (p25) and the easiest had up to 75.8% correct (p75).

Table 6 shows the themes of the 37 questions and the percentage of right/wrong answers for each question. Of the 37 questions, 13 had less than 50 per cent correct: questions 2, 3, 7, 10, 11, 12, 13, 15, 25, 27, 29, 30 and 35. These questions related to the following topics: swab technique, Unna boot, rest with elevated lower limbs for all types of chronic lower limb ulcers, topical antibiotics in colonised ulcers, systemic antibiotics, biofilm, critical colonisation, compressive therapy, cleaning ulcers, pressure relieving devices and knowledge about arterial ulcers.

The sentence with the highest number of correct answers was "Diabetic patients have a higher risk of neuropathic foot wounds" (97%); and the **sentence** with the lowest **number of correct answers was "Wounds with high exudation, an unpleasant odour and a greenish bed**

should be treated with systemic antibiotics" (10.8%).

Table 6: Distribution of the themes of the questions according to the percentage of correct answers and errors by nurses from the public health network in the municipality of Bauru, 2014.

Question topic	Hits %	Errors %	Don't know/Didn't answer %
Q1 - The best environment for healing	59,6	33,7	6,6
Q2 - Swab chronic wounds routinely	32,5	56,0	11,4
Q3 - Swab differentiates between colonised and infected wounds	16,9	67,5	15,7
Q4 - Hydrogel dressings	53,0	25,9	21,1
Q5 - Hydrocolloid dressings	63,9	24,1	12,0
Q6 - Activated carbon with silver	63,9	25,9	10,2
Q7 - Unna boot for arterial ulcers	45,2	39,2	15,7
Q8 - Braden Scale	75,3	3,6	21,1
Q9 - Diabetes and the risk of neuropathic wounds	97,0	2,4	0,6
Q10 - Chronic wounds and resting with the lower limbs elevated	45,2	46,4	8,4
Q11 - Indication for topical antibiotics in the treatment of colonised ulcers	49,4	33,7	16,9
Q12 - Biofilm	39,8	23,5	36,7
Q13 - Indication for systemic antibiotics	10,8	77,7	11,4
Q14 - Pressure ulcers	72,9	9,0	18,1
Q15 - Critical colonisation	12,7	75,3	12,0
Q16 - Clinic of plantar perforator disease	71,7	9,6	18,7
Q17 - Essential fatty acids	84,3	11,4	4,2
Q18 - Indication for mechanical debridement	83,7	13,3	3,0
Q19 - Knowledge of devitalised tissue and debridement	64,5	25,9	9,6
Q20 - Indication of compressive therapies	50,6	15,1	34,3
Q21 - Use of antiseptics for daily wound cleaning	59,6	32,5	7,8
Q22 - Knowledge about debridement of venous ulcers and PUs	77,7	13,9	8,4
Q23 - Knowledge of good granulation tissue	89,2	9,6	1,2
Q24 - Use of sterile gloves when dressing chronic wounds	53,6	44,0	2,4
Q25 - Occlusive dressings and compressive therapies	27,7	31,3	41,0
Q26 - Dressings for ulcers with a high degree of exudation	78,9	8,4	12,7
Q27 - Daily cleaning of wounds with soap and water	33,7	60,8	5,4
Q28 - Need for nutritional assessment in pressure ulcers	95,8	2,4	1,8
Q29 - Use of ring cushions for pressure ulcers	22,3	73,5	4,2
Q30 - Use of water-filled gloves in the prevention and treatment of pressure ulcers in the calcaneal region	34,9	59,0	6,0
Q31 - Plantar perforator disease and plantar load reduction	68,1	12,0	19,9
Q32 - Use of hospital mattresses as pressure reducing devices	84,3	11,4	4,2
Q33 - Cleaning wounds with 0.9% saline solution	88,6	10,2	1,2
Q34- Cleaning wounds with treated water	62,0	29,5	8,4
Q35 - Knowledge of potassium permanganate	41,6	22,9	35,5
Q36 - Use of sugar in colonised wounds	65,1	16,9	18,1
Q37 - Knowledge about arterial ulcers	72,9	7,2	19,9

The percentage of correct answers per specific topic in the knowledge questionnaire is shown in Table 7 and Graph 3. The highest median percentage of correct answers, at 79% (SD 27%), was in neuropathic ulcers; and the lowest, in clinical assessment (general assessment of the wound and concepts of colonisation and infection), with a median of 42% (SD 18%), with a statistically significant difference (**p<0**.05).

Table 7: Median percentage of correct answers per specific topic for nurses from the public health network in the municipality of Bauru, 2014.

Hits by Specific Subject		
	Average percentage of correct answers %	**Standard deviation %**
Pressure Ulcer (PU)	66,0	21,0
Venous and Arterial Ulcers	48,0	26,0
Neuropathic Ulcer	79,0	27,0
Clinical Assessment	42,0	18,0

Cleaning, Antisepsis and Debridement	61,0	21,0
Dressings	62,0	22,0
Total Hits General	58,0	15,0

There was no statistically significant association between the overall score of correct answers and length of time in the job (**p**= 0.78); length of time since graduation (**p**= 0.80); graduation institution, whether private or public (**p**= 0.78); whether or not they provided wound care (**p=0**.76); whether they were in a care or administrative role (**p=0**.61); how they considered training in wounds during graduation (**p**= 0.73); whether or not they did any refresher courses (**p**= 0.88).

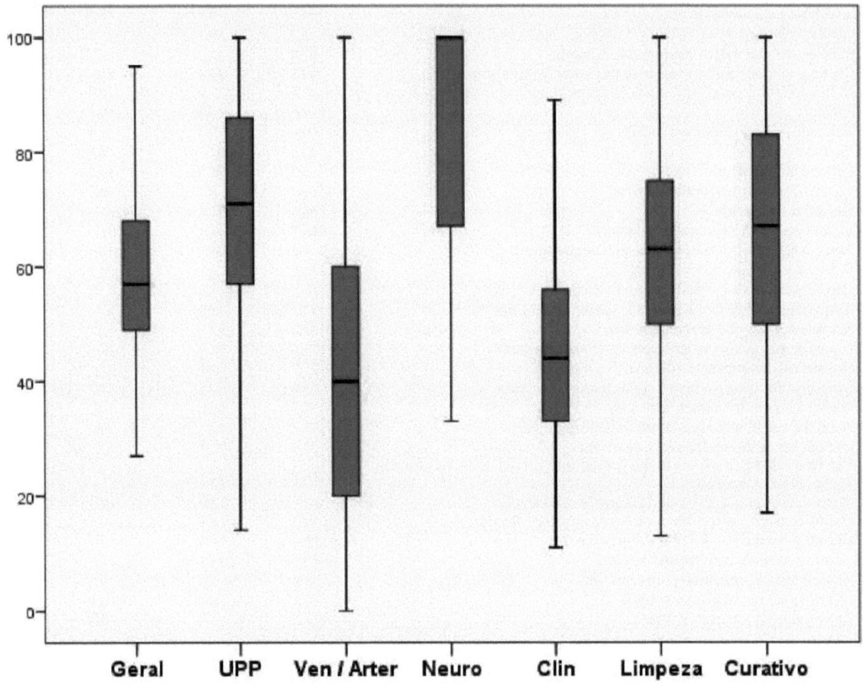

Graph 3: Box-plot with the median percentage of correct answers for specific topics, for nurses in the public health network in the municipality of Bauru, 2014.

There was an association between a better UPP score and nurses who performed the dressing (p=0.045; Graph 4).

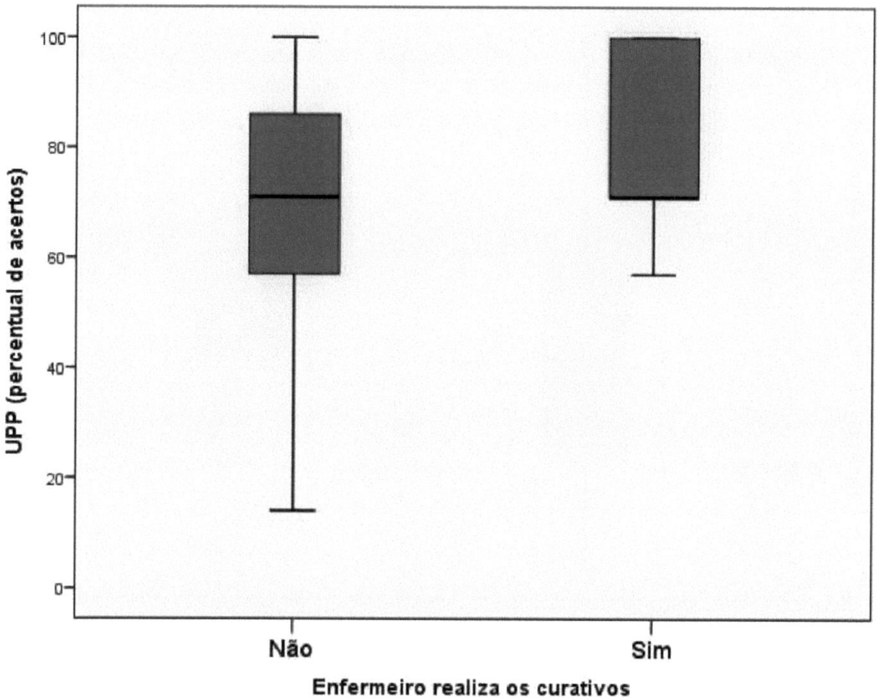

Graph 4: Box-plot with the median score of correct answers on topics related to pressure ulcers, regarding whether or not nurses from the public health network in the municipality of Bauru perform dressings, 2014.

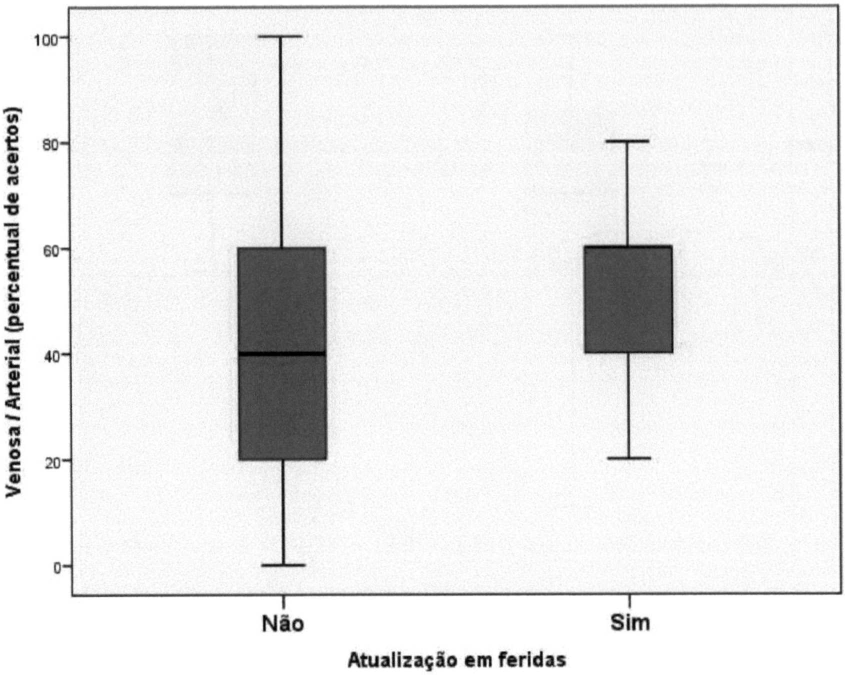

Graph 5: Box-plot with the median score of correct answers on topics related to venous and arterial ulcers, in relation to the update on wounds.

Nurses who answered that they keep up to date had a better score on topics related to venous and arterial ulcers (p=0.024; Graph 5); and those who carried out nursing consultations and prescribed dressings had a better score on topics related to cleaning, antisepsis and debridement (p=0.026; Graph 6).

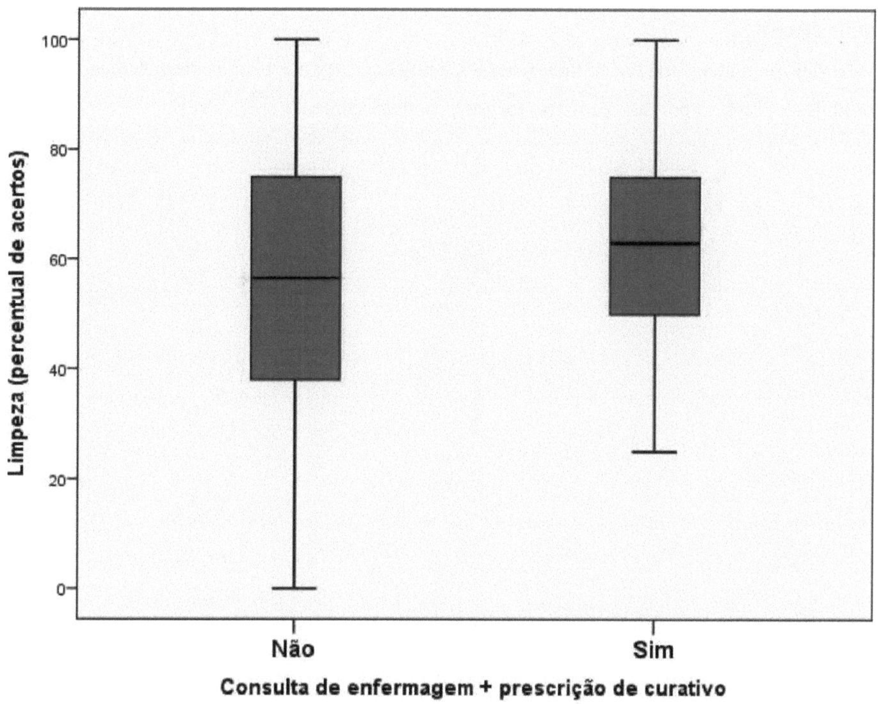

Graph 6: Box-plot showing the median number of correct answers on topics related to cleaning, antisepsis and debridement, considering nurses who carry out nursing consultations and prescribe dressings.

After studying the problems and verifying some aspects related to nurses' knowledge of wound care, a short thematic course was developed in a virtual environment: **"Update on wounds and dressings",** developed with the support of the Distance Education and Health Information Technology Centre (NEAD.TIS) of the Botucatu Medical School - Unesp.

This course will be made available free of charge to the health institutions in Bauru that took part in the research, and will be sent by email to participants who expressed a desire to receive feedback after the research has been finalised, and to health professionals in general who express an interest.

The course will last for a fixed period of 30 days, but it is up to the student to set a study timetable so that they can organise themselves. It consists of reading the content of the modules, video lessons, extra reading and a quiz to assess specific knowledge. The modules are divided into: Clinical assessment of wounds - general assessment of the wound and concepts of colonisation and infection; Concepts of cleaning **and debridement; Dressings; Approach** to pressure, venous, arterial and neuropathic ulcers.

In order for students to receive their Course Certificate, they must have completed and passed all the modules and take a pre- and post-test for each module studied.

CHAPTER 6

DISCUSSION

Caring for people with skin wounds is a daily practice for nurses working in primary care and/or hospital services. The nurse, among the members of the health team, plays an extremely important role in guiding, executing and supervising the nursing team in carrying out dressings, acting in prevention, assessment and indicating the appropriate treatment[60]. In this sense, and given the high prevalence of acute and chronic skin wounds, it is important that nurses in the healthcare network have the knowledge and technical skills to prevent, assess and treat these injuries.

Ferreira et al (2014)[10] emphasises that it is a constant challenge for nursing assistants or managers to obtain knowledge about the prevention and care of patients with wounds, as well as to keep up to date with evidence-based practice proposals. Keeping up to date with wounds results in better nursing care.

The main objective of this study was to identify whether nurses working in the public health network have knowledge about skin wounds, in line with best practices for caring for patients with these diseases, according to current scientific recommendations. In general, it can be identified that the participating nurses had a fair to good performance in the specific knowledge questionnaire, but many relevant topics had lower than desirable success rates.

Some sociodemographic data, training in skin wounds and clinical practice were studied to characterise the sample and to analyse possible interfering factors in knowledge on the subject.

As for the sociodemographic profile, the results confirmed that the profession is becoming more feminised, in line with other studies that have characterised nursing in Brazil. This is to be expected, given the historical association between caring and women's work[56,57,60]. However, men are entering the nursing profession, gradually changing this reality[56].

Age, time since graduation and time in practice show that most of the nurses are experienced. More than 90% of the participants graduated from private educational institutions in the region, showing that the region has a labour market capable of absorbing the workforce trained in the municipality.

Most of these professionals have care functions and participate in the hospital care network, mainly in the wards. The lower participation in the primary care network is justified by the greater number of nurses hired for the hospital network.

The majority of the participating nurses considered their training in wounds during their undergraduate studies to be fair to good, but when comparing the results of the specific questions, there was no greater number of correct answers among the nurses who declared that they had acquired better knowledge about wounds during their undergraduate studies. Only two Brazilian studies[56,57] were identified with the aim of investigating nursing students' knowledge of wound assessment and treatment.

In 2010, Santos et al[(56)] published a study carried out at the Health Sciences Centre of the Federal University of Paraíba, with 70 nursing students from the 8th and 9th periods. They concluded that the knowledge acquired during the course was insufficient for these students to be able to assess lesions in order to prescribe the appropriate behaviour for patients. Ferreira et al[57], in 2013, carried out a similar study with 68 undergraduate nursing students from the 9th period of the Public University of the State of Mato Grosso do Sul and the results showed that the level of knowledge about wound care is low and, therefore, investments in the undergraduate teaching of this course are necessary.

Other studies with similar objectives should be carried out in various Brazilian nursing teaching institutions, so that a real diagnosis can be made and proposals for curricular changes can be suggested, so that nursing graduates acquire sufficient knowledge for good practice in the treatment of cutaneous wounds.

Only 15.1 per cent of nurses answered that they did not provide any care to patients with wounds, a percentage identical to that of nurses with administrative functions, showing that nurses with care functions face the challenge of caring for patients with skin wounds in their daily lives.

Although they do, a considerable proportion of nurses do not update themselves on the subject in any way. Those who stated that they always keep up to date do so mainly informally, by seeking information from other nurses and consulting websites on the subject. Results also found by Ferreira et al (2014)[10] show that 80% of nurses only update themselves sometimes through periodicals and reading scientific articles.

The desirable forms of updating, such as reading scientific articles, congresses, symposia and extension courses, were less used. We can also see that a significant proportion of nurses update their knowledge using information from the pharmaceutical industry. Although this form of updating is not ideal, due to the undeniable conflicts of interest involved, the influence of these industries in encouraging and publicising new forms and technologies of wound treatment is notorious.[61]

It is desirable that professionals take a very critical look at all the information they obtain, whether from the pharmaceutical industry or by exchanging experiences with other nurses and doctors, as all these forms of updating have information biases. Improving the quality of care will only happen if there are opportunities for nurses and other professionals who care for people with wounds to take ongoing training courses[5].

This is a major challenge that must be taken on at different levels of care and by health managers within their remit. The lack of qualified professionals and training for the health team jeopardises the practice of care and meeting patients' needs.[60]

The vast majority of the participants in this study mentioned that, in everyday clinical practice, nurses do not perform the actual dressing of their patients; however, they are the nurses primarily responsible for prescribing this treatment. This reinforces the need for specific knowledge and updating for good practice in caring for patients with skin wounds and, consequently, reinforces the autonomy of nurses.

The nurse's duties include supervising the actions of the nursing team (assistants and technicians), drawing up the nursing care plan and guiding the care provided to patients. [7,10] It is the nurse's responsibility to regularly assess and document the skin of all patients under their care, so caution is needed when delegating this function to people who are not qualified. In this way, insufficient knowledge about wounds can have an impact on the care provided by nurses and other members of the nursing team.[10]

For this good care practice, there is also a need for dressing protocols, so that the best approach can be taken to patients, according to the best scientific evidence combined with the availability of existing resources in the institution. Only 62 per cent of the participating nurses answered that there were wound care protocols in their institution, thus highlighting the need to create and probably update specific protocols, respecting the particularities of the individual, the wound and also the institution. Similarly, in the results found by Ferreira et al (2014),[10] 34.3 per cent of nurses are unaware of the existence of protocols in the institutions where they work.

In a qualitative study with 14 nurses from four public hospitals in João Pessoa (PB), it was found that the lack of material leads to a superficial assessment of wounds; the absence of a protocol makes assessment difficult; and that medical imposition and lack of specific experience and training were the main difficulties revealed.[58]

The need to create material conditions and improve scientific knowledge in relation to the process of assessing and treating wounds has been highlighted.[58] Institutional dressing protocols allow for the systematisation of care for patients with wounds and make it possible to carry out the treatment and standardise the coverings used.[10]

The intersection of knowledge and resources available in the public healthcare network for wound treatment is not always desirable. The resources reported as being the best known and most used were collagenase, essential fatty acids and silver sulphadiazine. There is no evidence in the literature to support the use of these forms of local wound treatment[46,48], but they are probably the resources available in the institutions where the participating nurses work.

It is interesting to note that compression treatments for chronic venous ulcers, which are the most prevalent in the population,[36] are practically not used. This contradicts the study by Ferreira et al (2014)[10], in which the majority of respondents (57.1%) said they knew how to apply this therapy.

Compressive treatment, mainly Unna boots, elastic bands and multi-layer compression, are indispensable for this disease and the use of other local treatment resources, even high-tech ones, without compression, can be largely responsible for therapeutic failure, contributing to the chronicity of the wound, increased public and personal spending on ineffective treatments and consequences for the worsening quality of life of these patients.[35,41,42] Graduated compressive bandages in the distal region, from the foot to the knee, are standard treatment for venous ulcers without arterial involvement. It is therefore pertinent that nurses receive training in venous ulcer care, covering the assessment and application of these bandages.

Other resources considered more advanced for wound treatment and with some evidence for their indication[48], such as hydrocolloids and hydrogels, are known by the majority of nurses, but very little used. Other even more advanced technologies, such as hyperbaric oxygen therapy and negative pressure therapy, are used very little, although hyperbaric oxygen therapy is known by approximately 60 per cent of nurses. These results highlight the lack of investment or public management of the resources allocated to treating skin wounds.

As described in the methodology, the cognitive assessment of knowledge of topics related to the care of patients with wounds was carried out using questions prepared by two experts, and the answers were considered appropriate according to systematic reviews and specific, up-to-date guidelines.[45,46,48] The median score on this questionnaire was 5.6, however, most of the nurses obtained a good performance score and another significant proportion had a fair performance score.

In a recent study by Ferreira et al,[10] in 2014, on the knowledge and practice of nurses in caring for patients with wounds, carried out with 35 nurses from different sectors of a university hospital, the nurses obtained an average of 69.4% correct answers and concluded that the nurses had insufficient knowledge in some areas relating to the subject.

In this study, when assessing the number of correct answers to each of the 37 questions, 13 questions had less than 50% correct answers. The question with the lowest number of correct answers (10.8%) was question 13 (wounds with high exudation, an unpleasant odour and a greenish bed should be treated with systemic antibiotics). The correct answer to this question is "I don't agree", as the characteristics presented are not necessarily those of an infected ulcer, but of an ulcer with critical colonisation. According to current recommendations, systemic antibiotics are not indicated, as they do not show any improvement in ulcer healing, and local wound care is more indicated.[46,62]

Another question related to the same theme, colonisation/infection, which had a low hit rate (16.9%), was 3 (using the swab technique it is possible to differentiate colonised wounds from infected ones). The correct answer is "I don't agree", because the technique of collecting exudate from ulcers with a sterile swab from the depth of the ulcer, even after rigorous cleaning, does not guarantee that the cultures represent anything more than contaminating flora, with no predictivity for agents that may trigger skin, soft tissue or osteomyelitis infections, or to guide antibiotic therapy.

Considered the "gold standard" for wound culture samples, tissue **biopsy** identifies the microorganism infecting the tissue.[63] However, it is not a method available in all healthcare establishments.

The chronic wound has bacteria in its bed; whether a wound becomes infected depends especially on the individual's immunological resistance, as well as the microbial density and virulence.[63]

Despite their contraindication by experts,[64] swabs are still routinely used in primary care and hospital settings to guide the antimicrobial strategy in chronic ulcers, often only colonised, with no indication for systemic antibiotic treatment. Topical or systemic broad-spectrum antibiotic therapy contributes to the selection of resistant strains throughout the body, confers adverse effects and costs to the health system, and is not associated with higher healing rates if there is no patent infection.[65]

The question with the highest percentage of correct answers was 9 (Diabetic patients have a higher risk of neuropathic foot wounds), the answer to which was "I agree". Diabetes mellitus is a prevalent disease and neuropathic foot wounds are frequent complications.

Regarding the percentage of correct answers per specific topic, the lowest percentage was for venous and arterial ulcers and the highest percentages were for neuropathic ulcers and PUs. Venous and arterial ulcers are the main causes of chronic lower limb ulcers[24] and there is a pressing need for nurses and other professionals who provide care to these patients to seek knowledge. Neuropathic ulcers and PUs are also very prevalent and possible explanations for the higher rates of correct answers on these topics are that historically these injuries have been covered more frequently in the nursing field[66,67,68,69].

These results show that although the nurses' performance was generally good, there were some shortcomings in their knowledge of specific topics, mainly relating to the care of patients with venous and arterial ulcers and the concepts of colonisation and infection.

Curiously, the overall score of correct answers was not associated with any other variable, such as: length of time in the job; length of time since graduation; institution of graduation, whether private or public; place of work; whether or not they provided wound care; whether they were in a care or administrative role; how they considered training in wounds during graduation; and whether or not they did any refresher courses.

The fact that there was no association between better overall accuracy scores and being up-to-date on wounds is probably due to the way in which this updating was questioned: very broad, i.e. from exchanging information with other professionals to taking part in research groups and extension courses. As previously mentioned, some forms are not desirable and may have influenced this result.

However, there was an association between the score for specific topics and some variables. The score on the UPP theme was better for nurses who performed the dressing and those who performed the nursing consultation and prescribed the dressing had a better score on themes related to cleaning, antisepsis and debridement. These results may have been due to greater practical experience of these topics, as nurses who provide nursing consultations, prescribe and perform dressings are more likely to experience situations that stimulate the search for knowledge to solve care problems.

Nurses who answered that they keep up to date had a better score on topics related to venous and arterial ulcers, although knowledge deficits were detected in this area, given that the lowest percentage of correct answers was on this topic.

The lack of knowledge about skin wounds in the nursing field is not just a problem in Brazil, as several studies have shown the same deficiency in other countries.

Jones et al, in 2007,[70] in a study of different locations in the United States, to identify the consistency of chronic wound care practices with evidence-based recommendations for the treatment of venous, diabetic and pressure sores, concluded that practices were inconsistent with these recommendations.

In Spain, Pancorbo-Hidalgo et al, in 2007,[71] in a study on nurses' knowledge of UPP, concluded that although nurses are aware of many of the recommendations in the guidelines, there is insufficient knowledge and a low rate of implementation of some actions.

Barrett et al, 2009,[72] assessed Irish nurses' knowledge of lower limb wounds and concluded that, although many aspects were in line with the **guidelines**, there was a worrying lack of understanding of the fundamental concepts related to compressive therapy.

In 2010, Aydin and Karadag,[73] in a study of 243 nurses in Turkey, also on UPP, pointed out that the average correct score was 48.85 ± 11.99 out of 100 and concluded that nurses had insufficient knowledge in relation to the prevention and treatment of UPP.

The data analysed in this study shows the need for specific training for nurses in the prevention, assessment and treatment of the most prevalent skin wounds, as well as structuring healthcare units with the necessary human and material resources. They also suggest that care protocols need to be created and implemented by the teams involved in dealing with people with skin wounds, in order to guide effective prophylactic and therapeutic behaviour.

As a product of this research, we have developed a short thematic course on skin wounds in a virtual environment, with the aim of providing training for healthcare staff in a way that is easy to access outside of formal working hours. This course covers the main skin wounds, with an emphasis on current scientific recommendations for prevention and treatment.

This study has some limitations. Firstly, the size of the sample may have influenced the absence of some associations. There was a higher percentage of nurses from the hospital network, justified by the greater number of nurses hired in these services, but there would be a need to study a greater number of nurses from the primary network, in order to compare possible differences in practice and knowledge.

Another limitation is non-probability convenience sampling, which consists of selecting sample units that are more easily accessible. Therefore, nurses who were present at the time the researcher was in the unit to collect data and who were receptive to taking part in the study were invited.

Despite these limitations, the study was able to detect deficiencies in some of the practices recommended for wound care, such as: lack of protocols and non-compressible treatment for venous ulcers. A lack of knowledge was also detected, especially in relation to the concepts of critical colonisation and infection.

Ongoing, continuing and in-service education for nurses, aimed at training in its various possibilities, is essential for building and improving knowledge. In this context, this research does not exhaust the need for more in-depth studies on the subject, which could even subsidise new teaching proposals.

CHAPTER 7

CONCLUSIONS

The nurses who took part in the research were mainly female, with an average age of over 30 and a time since graduation and professional practice of around 10 years. Their degrees came mainly from private institutions in the municipality itself. Most of the nurses came from the hospital network and perform care functions.

A Training in skin wounds during undergraduate studies was judged to be fair or good. With regard to professional updating, most of the interviewees mentioned that they always or sometimes treat wounds, with a median time of 5 years, and more than 50 per cent said that they update themselves on the **subject of "wounds".**

The best known and most widely used therapeutic methods for wounds are collagenase ointment, essential fatty acids, silver sulphadiazine and neomycin. The Unna boot is well known and little used, while knowledge and use of negative pressure or vacuum therapy is still not widespread.

The nurses, in general, have regular knowledge on the subject of wounds, considering that the median score was 5.6. The topics with the highest levels of knowledge were neuropathic ulcers and UPP; and those with the lowest levels of knowledge were clinical assessment (general assessment of the wound and concepts of colonisation and infection).

N There was no association between correct answers and length of time in post, degree, degree institution, training in wounds during graduation, wound care, care or administrative role and professional updating.

Nurses who performed dressings scored better on PUs and those who kept up to date scored better on topics related to venous and arterial ulcers. Those who carried out nursing consultations and prescribed dressings scored better on topics related to cleaning, antisepsis and debridement.

E The need to train nurses in the field of wounds was highlighted, and a thematic short course (online) was designed to update health professionals in the care of patients with acute and chronic wounds.

CHAPTER 8

REFERENCES

1 Ferreira AM, Bogamil DDD, Tormena PC. Nurses and wound care: in search of autonomous care. Arq ciências da saúde 2008; **15**: 105-9.

2 Ferreira AM, Candido MCFS, Candido MA. The care of patients with wounds and the construction of nurses' autonomy. Rev enferm UERJ 2010; **18**: 656-60.

3 Federal Nursing Council (Br) Resolution 311/2007. Approves the reformulation of the Code of Ethics for nursing professionals. Rio de Janeiro: COFEn; 2007. .

4 Leadebal ODCP, Filho WDF, Nóbrega MML, Galdino TB. Analysis of the didactic-pedagogical bases for teaching the systematisation of nursing care. Rev *Min Enferm* 2009; **13**: 64-75.

5 Kobayashi RM, Leite MMJ. Developing nurses' professional competences in service. Rev. Bras. Enferm. 2010; **63**: 243-9.

6 Brazil. Ministry of Education. Department of Higher Education. Curriculum Guidelines for Undergraduate Programmes. Resolution CNE/ CES N° 3. http://portal.mec.gov.br/cne/arquivos/pdf/CES03.pdf (accessed Jan 5, 2015).

7 COFEN. Decree 94.406/87. Regulates Law n° 7.498, of 25 June 1987. 1986, which provides for the practice of Nursing, and makes other provisions. http://www.cofen.gov.br/decreto-n-9440687_4173.html. (accessed Dec 20, 2014).

8 Borges EL, Saar SRC, Lima VLAN. Subsidies for protocol construction. In: Borges EL, Saar SRC, Magalhães MBB, Gomes FSL, Lima VLAN, eds. Wounds: how to treat, 2nd edn. Belo Horizonte - MG: Editora Coopmed Ltda, 2008: 1-13.

9 Dutton M, Chiarella M, Curtis K. The role of the wound care nurse: an integrative review. *Br J Community Nurs* 2014; **Suppl**: S39-40, S42-7.

10 Ferreira AM, Rigotti MA, Barcelos LS, Simão CMF, Ferreira DN, Gonçalves RQ. Knowledge and practice of nurses on care for patients with wounds. Rev *pesqui Cuid fundam* 2014; **6**: 1178-90.

11 Abbade LPF. Ulcerative disorders. In: Belda Jr W, di Chiacchio N, Criado PR, eds. Treatise on Dermatology, 2nd edn. São Paulo: Atheneu Rio, 2014: 80330.

12 Abbade LPF. Differential Diagnoses of Chronic Ulcers of the Lower Limbs. In: Malagutti, W; Kakihara CT, ed. Dressings, stomas and dermatology: a professional approach. São Paulo: Martinari, 2009: 77-93.

13 Saar SRC, Lima VLAN. Assessment of people with wounds. In: Borges EL, Saar SRC, Magalhães MBB, Gomes FSL, Lima VLAN, eds. Wounds: how to treat them. Belo Horizonte - MG, 2007: 55-77.

14 Iron GL. Wound assessment. In: Iron GL, ed. Wounds: new approaches, clinical management

and atlas in colour, 2nd edn. Rio de Janeiro: Guanabara Koogan Ltda, 2010: 143-56.

15 Borges EL. Care for patients with complex surgical wounds. In: Borges EL, Saar SRC, Magalhães MBB, Gomes FS, Lima VLAN, eds. Wounds: how to treat them. Belo Horizonte - MG: Editora Coopmed Ltda, 2008: 95-112.

16 **Mandelbaum SH, Pampado di Santis É, SanfAna Mandelbaum MH.** Scarring: Current concepts and auxiliary resources - Part II. An. Bras. Dermatol. 2003; **78**: 525-42.

17 Saar SRC. Considerations on wound infections. In: Borges EL, Saar SRC, Magalhães MBB, Gomes FSL, Lima VLAN, eds. Wounds: how to treat, 2nd edn. Belo Horizonte - MG: Editora Coopmed Ltda, 2008: 79-94.

18 Abbade LPF. Wound bed preparation. In: Malaguti W, Kakihara CT, eds. Dressings, Stomas and Dermatology, 1st edn. São Paulo: Martinari, 2009: 6376.

19 Pannier F, Rabe E. Differential diagnosis of leg ulcers. Phlebology 2013; **28 Suppl 1**: 55-60.

20 McCulloch J, Mahoney E, McCallon S. Enhancing the Role of Physical Therapy in Venous Leg Ulcer Management. JAMA dermatology 2014; published online Dec 17. DOI:10.1001/jamadermatol.2014.4042.

21 Jockenhofer F, Gollnick H, Herberger K, et al. Aetiology, comorbidities and cofactors of chronic leg ulcers: retrospective evaluation of 1 000 patients from 10 specialised dermatological wound care centres in Germany. Int Wound J 2014; published online Dec 5. DOI:10.1111/iwj.12387.

22 Maffei FH, Magaldi C, Pinho SZ, et al. Varicose veins and chronic venous insufficiency in Brazil: prevalence among 1755 inhabitants of a country town. Int J *Epidemiol* 1986; **15**: 210-7.

23 Valencia IC, Falabella A, Kirsner RS, Eaglstein WH. Chronic venous insufficiency and venous leg ulceration. J Am *Acad Dermatol* 2001; **44**: 40121; quiz 422^.

24 Grey JE, Harding KG, Enoch S. Venous and arterial leg ulcers. *BMJ Br Med J* 2006; **332**: 347-50.

25 Reddy M. Pressure ulcers. *Clin Evid (Online)* 2011; **5**: 1901.

26 Gardiner JC, Reed PL, Bonner JD, Haggerty DK, Hale DG. Incidence of hospital-acquired pressure ulcers - a population-based cohort study. *Int Wound J* 2014; published online Dec 3. DOI:10.1111/iwj.12386.

27 Rogenski NMB, Santos VLCG. Study on the incidence of pressure ulcers in a university hospital. Rev *Latinoam Enferm* 2005; **13**: 474-80.

28 Gomes FSL, Bastos MAR, Matozinhos FP, Temponi HR, Velásquez-Meléndez G. Factors associated with pressure ulcers in patients admitted to Adult Intensive Care Centres. Rev *da Esc Enferm* 2010; **44**: 10706.

29 Boulton AJM. Diabetic neuropathy and foot complications. *Handb Clin Neurol* 2014; **126**: 97-107.

30 Nascimento OJM. Leprosy neuropathy: clinical presentations. *Arq Neuropsiquiatr* 2013; **71**: 661-6.

31 Rosero, A C Gonzalez P V, Nery, J A C Mendonça IRSM, Azulay RD. Perforating plantar malunion: a study of 50 cases. An *Acad Nac Med* 1996; **156**: 5-8.

32 Baba M, Davis WA, Davis TME. A longitudinal study of foot ulceration and its risk factors in community-based patients with type 2 diabetes: the Fremantle Diabetes Study. *Diabetes Res Clin Pract* 2014; **106**: 42-9.

33 Abbade LPF, Lastoria S, Rollo HD, Stolf HO. A sociodemographic, clinical study of patients with venous ulcer. *Int J Dermatol* 2005; **44**: 989-92.

34 Herber OR, Schnepp W, Rieger MA. A systematic review on the impact of leg **ulceration on patients' quality of life.** *Health Qual Life Outcomes* 2007; **5**: 44.

35 Meissner MH. Venous ulcer care: which dressings are cost effective? *Phlebol J Venous Dis* 2014; **29**: 174-80.

36 Etufugh CN, Phillips TJ. Venous ulcers. *Clin Dermatol* 2007; **25**: 121-30.

37 Bergman-Evans B, Cuddigan J, Bergstrom N. Clinical practice guidelines: prediction and prevention of pressure ulcers. *Todays OR Nurse* 2001; **16**: 3340.

38 Apelqvist J, Ragnarson-Tennvall G, Persson U, Larsson J. Diabetic foot ulcers in a multidisciplinary setting. An economic analysis of primary healing and healing with amputation. J *Intern Med* 1994; **235**: 463-71.

39 Bild DE, Selby J V., Sinnock P, Browner WS, Braveman P, Showstack JA. Lower-extremity amputation in people with diabetes. Epidemiology and prevention. *Diabetes Care* 1989; **l2**: 24-31.

40 Zimmet SE. Venous leg ulcers: modern evaluation and management. *Dermatol Surg* 1999; **25**: 236-41.

41 **O'Meara S, Cullum NA, Nelson EA. Compression for venous leg ulcers.** *Cochrane Database Syst Rev* 2009; : CD000265.

42 **Annells M, O'Neill J, Flowers C. Compression bandaging for venous leg ulcers:** The essentialness of a willing patient. *J Clin Nurs* 2008; **17**: 350-9.

43 Abbade LPF, Lastória S. Approach to patients with venous leg ulcers. An. Bras. Dermatol. 2006; **81**: 509-22.

44 Zamboni P, Cisno C, Marchetti F, *et al.* Minimally invasive surgical management of primary venous ulcers vs. compression treatment: a randomised clinical trial. 2003.

45 Steed DL, Attinger C, Colaizzi T, *et al.* Guidelines for the treatment of diabetic ulcers. Wound Repair Regen. 2006; **14**: 680-92.

46 Bolton LL, Girolami S, Corbett L, van Rijswijk L. The Association for the Advancement of Wound Care (AAWC) venous and pressure ulcer guidelines. *Ostomy Wound Manage* 2014;

60: 24-66.

47 Falabella AF. Debridement and wound bed preparation. Dermatol. Ther. 2006; **19**: 317-25.

48 Chaby G, Senet P, Vaneau M, *et al.* Dressings for acute and chronic wounds: a systematic review. *Arch Dermatol* 2007; **143**: 1297-304.

49 Kamolz LP, Wild T. Wound bed preparation: The impact of debridement and wound cleansing. *Wound Med* 2013; **1**: 44-50.

50 Pullen R, Popp R, Volkers P, Fusgen I. Prospective randomised double-blind study of the wound-debriding effects of collagenase and fibrinolysin/deoxyribonuclease in pressure ulcers. *Ageing* 2002; **31**: 12630.

51 Westerhof W, van Ginkel CJ, Cohen EB, Mekkes JR. Prospective randomised study comparing the debriding effect of krill enzymes and a non-enzymatic treatment in venous leg ulcers. 1990.

52 Vig S, Dowsett C, Berg L, et al. Evidence-based recommendations for the use of negative pressure wound therapy in chronic wounds: Steps towards an international consensus. J. Tissue Viability. 2011; 20.
DOI:10.1016/j.jtv.2011.07.002.

53 Sibbald RG, Orsted H, Schultz GS, Coutts P, Keast D. Preparing the wound bed 2003: focus on infection and inflammation. Ostomy Wound Manage 2003; 49: 23-51.

54 Elizabeth A Ayello, Keryln Carville, Jacqui Fletcher, David Keast, David Leaper, Christina Lindholm, José Luis Lázaro Martínez, Silindile Mavanini, Inkosi Albert Luthuli Andrew McBain, Zena Moore, Supaporn Opasanon, Elaine Pina. International consensus. Appropriate use of silver dressings in wounds. An expert working group consensus. 2012.

55 Smart V, Alavi A, Coutts P, et al. Contact allergens in persons with leg ulcers: a Canadian study in contact sensitisation. Int J Low Extrem Wounds 2008; 7: 120-5.

56 Santos AAR, Medeiros ABA, Soares MJGO CM. Assessment and treatment of wounds: the knowledge of nursing students. Rev enferm UERJ 2010; 18: 547-52.

57 Ferreira AM, Rigotti MA, Pena SB, Paula DS, Ramos IB, Sasaki VDM. Knowledge and practice of nursing students on wound care. Esc *Anna Nery* 2013; 17: 211-9.

58 Morais GF da C, Oliveira SH dos S, Soares MJGO. Assessment of wounds by nurses in public hospital institutions. Texto Context. - Enferm. 2008; 17: 98-105.59 Hora HRM, Rego GT, Arica J.
Reliability in Quality Questionnaires: A Study with Cronbach's Alpha Coefficient. *Prod Produção* 2010; 11: 85-103.

60 Azevedo IC, Costa RKS, Holanda CSM, Salvetti MG, Torres G V. Knowledge of Family Health Strategy Nurses on the Evaluation and Treatment of Oncological Wounds. *Rev Bras Cancerol* 2014; 60: 119-27.

61 Palma A, Vilaça MM. Conflicts of interest in the research, production and dissemination of medicines. História, Ciências, Saúde-Manguinhos. 2012; 19: 919-32.

62 O'Meara S, Al-Kurdi D, Ologun Y, Ovington LG, Martyn-St James M, Richardson R. Antibiotics and antiseptics for venous leg ulcers. *Cochrane Database Syst Rev* 2014; 1: CD003557.

63 Souza JM, Vieira ÉC, Cortez TM, Mondelli AL, Miot HA, Abbade LPF. Clinical and microbiological evaluation of chronic leg ulcers: a cross-sectional study. *Adv Skin Wound Care* 2014; 27: 222-7.

64 Bonham PA. Swab cultures for diagnosing wound infections: a literature review and clinicai guideline. J *Wound Ostomy Continence Nurs;* ***36:*** 389-95.

66 Moreira RC, Sales CA. Nursing care for diabetic foot patients: a phenomenological approach. *Rev Esc Enferm USP* 2010; ***44***: 896-903.

67 Pereira SVM, Bachion MM, Souza AGC de, Vieira SMS. Leprosy evaluation: an experience report by nursing students. Rev. Bras. Enferm. 2008; **61**: 774-80.

68 Freitas CASL, Silva Neto AV da, Ximenes Neto FRG, Albuquerque IMN, Cunha ICKO. Nursing consultation with leprosy patients in the territory of the Family Health Strategy: perceptions of nurses and patients. Rev. Bras. Enferm. 2008; **61**: 757-63.

69 Alves AR, Belaz K, Rodrigues RM, Ribeiro SMT, Kato TTM, Medina NVJ. The importance of nursing care in preventing pressure ulcers in hospitalised patients. Rev *Inst Ciênc Saúde* 2008; **26**: 397-402.

70 Jones KR, Fennie K, Lenihan A. Evidence-based management of chronic wounds. Adv *Skin Wound Care* 2007; **20**: 591-600.

71 Pancorbo-Hidalgo PL, García-Fernández FP, López-Medina IM, López-Ortega **J. Pressure ulcer care in Spain: Nurses' knowledge and clinical practice.** J Adv *Nurs* 2007; **58**: 327-38.

72 Barrett S, Cassidy I, Graham MM. National survey of Irish community nurses leg ulcer management practices and knowledge. J *Wound Care* 2009; **18**: 1812, 184,186 passim.

73 **Aydin AK, Karadag A. Assessment of Nurses' Knowledge and Practice in** Prevention and Management of Deep Tissue Injury and Stage I Pressure Ulcer. *J Wound Ostomy Cont Nurs* 2010; **37**: 487-94.

MIX
Papier aus verantwortungsvollen Quellen
Paper from responsible sources
FSC® C105338

Printed by Books on Demand GmbH, Norderstedt / Germany